The Guide To Staying Healthy

After 40 For Men...

The Keta Way

You can also follow me here on Facebook

https://www.facebook.com/Staying-fit-after-40-112856910143415/

to stay updated with our latest news and new book releases.

Table of Contents

Summary

A Ketogenic diet is a diet with very low carbohydrate compensated by a lipid reinforcement. The metabolized fat creates a state of nutritional ketosis. The ketogenic diet is a diet rich in lipids particularly fashionable for some years. As men age, their nutritional needs change. Your ability to burn calories decreases with age, which is why the amount of food you need is likely to be reduced, or you will experience a decrease in appetite. Aging also means that the amount of vitamins and minerals you need to be healthy is likely to differ from what you needed when you were young.

Your body may have difficulty absorbing certain nutrients in foods such as calcium, iron and vitamin B12. Ask your doctor or a registered dietitian for advice. To stay healthy, you must make choices in accordance with Canada's Food Guide. Stock up on fruits and vegetables, whole grains, low-fat dairy products, and opt for fibre-rich alternatives to meat, such as beans and lentils. By making healthy food choices, being physically active and not smoking, you can avoid many chronic diseases and live longer in good health.

- The body changes as you get older.
- As men age, their nutritional needs change.
- Your ability to burn calories decreases with age.
- You can avoid many chronic diseases and live longer in good health by making healthy food choices, being physically active and not smoking.
- The ketogenic diet is a way of life rather than a limited-duration diet. It is not supposed to be abandoned after a few months.
- A keto diet refers to a ketogenic diet, which is a high protein diet and low in carbohydrates. The goal is to get more calories from protein and fat than carbohydrates.
- Despite the benefits it can have, the ketogenic diet is not perfect.
- Once adapted to ketosis, it becomes rarer that one feels hunger.
- The hunger-cutting side of this diet is very important. It becomes slimming to the extent that it is easier to resist the temptation of snacking.

CHAPTER 1

RESERVED FOR MEN - STAYING HEALTHY AT 40

The fact that the body changes as you get older is not a secret. However, you can facilitate the process by taking care of your body. Stay healthy longer! Follow these tips to learn how to combat the health problems that men face as they get older.

NUTRITION AND AGING

As men age, their nutritional needs change. Your ability to burn calories decreases with age, which is why the amount of food you need is likely to be reduced, or you will experience a decrease in appetite. Aging also means that the amount of vitamins and minerals you need to be healthy is likely to differ from what you needed when you were young. Your body may have difficulty absorbing certain nutrients in foods such as calcium, iron and vitamin B12. Ask your doctor or a registered dietitian for advice.

MEN'S HEALTH ISSUES TO CONSIDER

Smoking cigarettes, not exercising, and making inappropriate food choices are some of the most common reasons people get sick, especially as they get older. Fortunately, it's still time for you to make some healthy changes! The following four health problems commonly affect men when they reach their fifties. For each of them, you will find suggestions on how to "increase" or "decrease" in order to stay in good health longer.

1.　　　**Heart disease**

This is a term which consists of several different conditions which affect your heart and arteries. This condition includes heart attacks, chest pains and arterial occlusion etc. To reduce the risk of heart disease, choose:

To increase:

- fatty fish rich in omega-3 fatty acids (salmon, trout). Try to eat twice a week;
- the fibres, consuming whole grains, beans, as well as fruit and vegetables;
- the healthy fats, such as olive oil or canola oil and margarine trans-fat;
- Healthy fats, such as canola oil, olive oil and trans-fat.
- unsalted nuts, ¼ cup (60 ml) five times a week;
- the exercise, to practice 30 to 60 minutes most days of the week;

And decrease:

- the saturated fat contained butter, cheese and fatty meats;
- the trans fats found in hydrogenated oils (shortening, hard margarines), and processed foods from fast food;
- salty foods;
- the cigarettes;
- alcohol (no more than two glasses a day).

2.   Prostate cancer

This is the most common type of cancer in older men. It affects the prostate gland, which is an organ of the male reproductive system. To reduce the risk of prostate cancer, choose:

To increase:

- lycopene is an antioxidant; it is found in tomatoes and cooked tomato products. Examples are juice, tomato paste and soup;
- selenium, a mineral found in Brazil nuts, whole grains and meat;
- fruits and vegetables;
- the legumes (chickpeas, beans, lentils) and soy;

And decrease:

- calcium: Make sure you have adequate daily calcium intake (1200 mg), but not more. Although calcium is essential for keeping bones strong, eating too much (over 1500 mg / day) can increase the risk of prostate cancer.

3.   Drop

Gout is a form of arthritis caused by the presence of a very high level of uric acid in the blood. It also causes joint pain and increases the risk of formation of kidney stones. You can follow these steps to avoid gout:

To increase:

- low-fat dairy products at three servings per day;
- fibre, contained in whole grains, beans, as well as fruits and vegetables;
- the vitamin C present in peppers, citrus fruits, broccoli, and strawberries;
- the folic acid, as found in the beans, whole grains, almonds and asparagus;
- the exercise;

And decrease:

- foods rich in "purine", such as:
- fish: anchovies, sardines, herring, trout, salmon
- the shrimp
- offal
- soy
- dried mushrooms;
- red meats (beef, pork, lamb), limited to a portion of 75 g (2.5 oz.);
- the alcohol, in particular beer. Just one drink a day.

4.   Osteoporosis

A disease that results in weakening and thinning of the bones, as well as a decrease in bone volume. Many people think that this is a "typical female disease", but it can also affect men. To reduce the risk of osteoporosis, choose:

To increase:

- the calcium and vitamin D;
- exercise, to keep bones strong;
- vitamin B12 supplements, if your intake is insufficient (talk to your doctor);

And decrease:

- the alcohol. Limit yourself to two glasses daily;
- the salty food. Be sure to consume less than 1500 mg of sodium daily.

To stay healthy, you must make choices in accordance with Canada's Food Guide. Stock up on fruits and vegetables, whole grains, low-fat dairy products, and opt for fibre-rich alternatives to meat, such as lentils and beans. Being physically active, choosing healthy food choices and avoid smoking can make you live longer and help you avoid chronic diseases.

CHAPTER 2

HEALTH CHECK UP AT THE AGE OF 40

SCREENING FOR CANCERS AGED 40 TO 49

The three most common cancers in men are cancers of the prostate, bronchial and colorectal. The risk of developing one of these cancers increases with age, but fifty years is the age at which their incidence rates increase significantly. It is therefore from this threshold that the recommendations agree to offer screening to men at medium risk. From age 40 to 49, screening recommendations are a gray area and are often less well known. Below age 40, the incidence of these three forms of cancer is very low. For the three most common cancers in humans, here are the recommendations for early detection, before age 50.

1.   Colorectal cancer

In Switzerland, colorectal cancer (CRC) in humans is the third most common type of cancer in terms of frequency and mortality. For the general population (at medium risk), the US Preventive Services Task Force (USPSTF) strongly recommends (type A recommendation) colorectal screening of 40 to 75 years. From age 76 to age 84, screening is done on an individual basis because the risk / benefit profile of this age group no longer justifies routine screening (type C recommendation). Beyond age 84, screening is not recommended (Type D recommendation). Before age 50, colonoscopy screening is only recommended in high-risk patients. About a quarter of cancers are diagnosed in these. Without discussing hereditary syndromic cancers (the most common of which are Lynch syndrome, familial adenomatous polyposis, called classical or attenuated polyposis, MUTYH-associated polyposis and CRC familial X syndrome) which concern the youngest, with screening generally proposed between 10 and 25 years, according to the syndrome.

2.   Prostate cancer

Prostate cancer is the most common cancer in men. According to the FOPH, one in six men will develop one (16.4%). According to the FSO, the incidence between 2008 and 2012 for the 40-44 age group was 7/6236 cases (0.11%) while it was 1395/6236 (22%) for the 65-69 years. Recall that the USPSTF recommends not to screen for this cancer by the prostate specific antigen (PSA) assay (type D recommendation), while other medical societies emphasize the decision process shared with, from this is an individualized screening decision. We summarize in a table the recommendations for this cancer before age 50.

3.   Pulmonary cancer

In humans, bronchial cancer is the second most common cancer and is the leading cause of death due to cancer. According to the SFSO, between 2008 and 2012, the incidence of this cancer was highest in the 65-69 age group (17.7%) and 3.7% in the 40-49 age group. The two largest randomized controlled studies, the NLST (National Lung Screening Trial) in the United States, published in 2011, and the European study NELSON (Dutch-Belgian Randomized Lung Cancer Screening Trial), for which the results are expected in 2016, did not include any patient under 50 years of age. Following the release of the NLST results, all US medical societies recommend chest cancer screening at low doses in high-risk patients at the earliest age of 50 years. There is no recommendation on screening for bronchial cancer in men under 50 years of age. The setting up of this screening in Switzerland is discussed elsewhere by Guessous and Cornuz, who stress that the criteria for inclusion of patients should be the same as those of the NLST.

CHAPTER 3

•••●•••

SCREENING FOR CARDIOVASCULAR DISEASES BETWEEN 40 AND 45 YEARS

Primary prevention recommendations for cardiovascular events are based on scores that define the risk of occurrence of such events. In practice, the two most used and best adapted scores for cardiovascular prevention in Switzerland are the PROCAM 12 score and the SCORE. Age is used as a measure of cardiovascular risk exposure time, rather than as a risk factor per se. It reflects the duration of exposure of an individual to other risk factors. It appears that men under 50 have an absolute risk of cardiovascular mortality that remains low (0-2%), even when the risk factors are unfavourable. It is interesting to note that the absolute risk of 10-year cardiovascular mortality in a 40-year-old man with high blood pressure and systolic blood pressure of 180 mmHg and a total cholesterol level of 8 mmol / l is identical to that of a 65-year-old non-smoking man with a systolic blood pressure of 120 mmHg and a total cholesterol level of 4 mmol / l, i.e. 2%.

SEXUALLY TRANSMITTED INFECTIONS BETWEEN 40 AND 49 YEARS

Men are not the most affected by sexually transmitted infections (STIs), but the incidence in this group is increasing according to the Centres for Disease Control and Prevention (CDC). Risk factors should guide us to offer STI testing, but age is not one of them. Young men as well as middle-aged men, with identical risk factors, should have similar STI screening. Let's not forget the incidence of major STIs according to the FOPH: men between 25 and 34 years are most often affected by HIV (in men who have sex with men), chlamydia and gonorrhoea (regardless of their age). sexual preferences); those between 35 and 44 years old with syphilis and HIV (among heterosexuals).

ANDROPAUSE AND SUBSTITUTION IN TESTOSTERONE

Aging is associated with a slow decrease in testicular testosterone production in humans, usually 1-2% per year. Andropause, or hypogonadism in older men (LOH or late-onset hypogonadism of), is defined by a lower rate of testosterone at 8 nmol/L (or between 8 and 11 nmol/L with a lower free testosterone levels at 220 pmol/l), accompanied by a triad of sexual symptoms: erectile dysfunction, decreased libido and decreased morning erections. In Europe, the prevalence of andropause among men increases from 0.15 to 5.1% between 40 and 79 years. Beyond aging, we know that certain factors such as smoking and weight influence testosterone levels: andropause is for example associated in 73% of cases with overweight or obesity. This suggests that hormonal decline could be reduced with the management of health and lifestyle. There is no certainty about the consequences of lowering testosterone levels with age. Several elements suggest that the decline of serum testosterone may be the cause of several effects of aging in humans, including decreased sexual function, fatigue, decreased muscle strength, mood disorders, decreased density bone mineral. 16Testosterone substitution remains controversial in terms of indication and administration pattern. The US Food and Drug Administration concluded that the beneficial effects of testosterone administration could not be well demonstrated and that the substitute products were only approved for men with low testosterone levels secondary to causes. identified. It is also crucial to take into account the possible side effects of a substitution before starting it, including the aggravation of testosterone-related diseases, particularly in the prostate.

CHAPTER 4

KETOGENIC DIET: EVERYTHING YOU NEED TO KNOW

In recent decades, many low carb diets have emerged but there is one that is gaining popularity: the ketogenic diet. Far from being a trend of the moment, this diet was already practiced in the 1920s in clinics to treat patients who are overweight, sick and have epilepsy.

WHAT IS THE KETOGENIC DIET?

The ketogenic diet is a very high fat and low carbohydrate diet that has many benefits: constant weight loss, increased energy, improved cognitive abilities, hormonal balance and reduced risk of chronic diseases such as hyperglycemia, hypertension or high triglyceride levels. When you follow a ketogenic diet, your body reaches the metabolic state of ketosis:

- Glucose, derived from foods rich in carbohydrates and a fast source of energy, decreases drastically.
- The body will have to find other sources of energy.

- It will burn more fat and produce larger amounts of ketones, small molecules that contribute to energy metabolism.

In order to achieve the metabolic status of ketosis and stay there, at least 75% of your daily calories must come from fat so that your body can produce ketone bodies that will maintain your energy level. In the absence of carbohydrates and glucose, your body will have to tap into the fats from your diet and into your fat stores to produce energy, which will promote weight loss.

SOME TIPS TO GET THE MOST FROM THE KETOGENIC DIET:

1.   USE FAT FROM FOOD AND UNPROCESSED

To prevent or reverse signs of poor health, I recommend a comprehensive approach to the ketogenic diet. This means that most of your calories must come from healthy, unprocessed, high fat ketogenic foods:

- olive and coconut oil
- ghee (clarified butter)
- avocado
- nuts
- oily fish and foods from pasture fed animals such as butter, eggs or meat.

Avoid at all costs foods such as processed meats (bacon or salami), poor quality meats from industrial farms, processed cheeses, fish from farms, foods stuffed with synthetic additives and refined vegetable oils (canola, safflower and sunflower oil). Even though they are all high in fat, they can have adverse health effects.

1. DO NOT FORGET THE VEGETABLES!

Eat lots of green and non-floury vegetables as they contain important vitamins, minerals, fibre and antioxidants. Try to include a handful or two of them at each meal. Just make sure to limit or eliminate mealy vegetables such as potatoes, beets or squash, which are too rich in carbohydrates.

2. DO NOT OVERDO WITH PROTEINS

One of the factors that makes the ketogenic diet very different from other low carb diets is the fact that it advocates consuming less protein and more fat. It includes moderate amounts of protein (about 15% of daily calories), while carbohydrates are limited to 5 or 10% of calorie intake (or about 25 to 35 grams per day).

To note: It is important to eat the right amount of macronutrients because it will allow you to reach the state of ketosis and produce ketone bodies, essential for good mental and physical health despite a strict restriction of carbohydrates. If you eat too much protein, it may become glucose, which is counterproductive to the ketogenic diet and will prevent you from getting to the state of ketosis.

3. TRY INTERMITTENT FASTING

Fasting has a very positive impact on hormones, blood sugar regulation, inflammation and detoxification. Intermittent fasting is a strategy that can help you maximize the results of your ketogenic diet. Fasting and the ketogenic diet combine perfectly because the ketone bodies produced have the effect of reducing appetite, which facilitates long periods without eating. Fasting helps in regulating ghrelin and leptin, the hormones of hunger, while having beneficial effects on insulin sensitivity and weight loss. You can do intermittent fasting by limiting the periods during which you eat at 4 to 9 o'clock windows (so you will fast for 15 to

20 hours). You can also try alternating fasting which consists of restricting your calorie intake by 75% once or twice a week.

4. HYDRATE YOURSELF AND CONSUME ENOUGH ELECTROLYTES

During a ketogenic diet, do not forget to drink enough water and other healthy drinks (herbal teas, squeezed juices, organic coffee, green tea and bone broth). Also remember to consume salt to provide your body with enough potassium, magnesium and other electrolytes. Use sea salt or pink salt from the Himalayas to season your dishes or drink salted broths. The electrolytes will not only promote your digestion, have a beneficial effect on the muscular and cellular functions, your sleep, your morale and give you energy.

To note: While the ketogenic diet differs considerably from other low fat diets, it is generally considered to be health friendly for most people who practice it. But beware, it is always recommended to consult your doctor before starting a ketogenic diet. In particular, people with diabetes, eating disorders, liver or kidney problems or any other genetic deficiency that could interfere with fat absorption, as well as pregnant or breastfeeding women should not practice the ketogenic diet.

TEMPORARY SIDE EFFECTS OF THE KETOGENIC DIET

Some people may also experience side effects of the ketogenic diet (headache, lack of energy, food cravings, weakness or confused brain) during the transition phase but these symptoms usually disappear after 1 to 2 weeks.

CHAPTER 5

KETOGENIC DIET

The ketogenic diet or ketogenic diet is a diet with very low carbohydrate compensated by a lipid reinforcement. The metabolized fat creates a state of nutritional ketosis. It is a diet rich in lipids which was particularly fashionable for a few years. It has been used for over a hundred years to treat certain pathologies including epilepsy. Keto diet aims to reduce the consumption of carbohydrates in favour of lipids to cause state of ketosis. Apart from weight loss, it has many health benefits.

The ketogenic diet prescribes a diet low in carbohydrates, compensated by a reinforcement of lipids. Fat intake significantly reduces carbohydrate requirements. Fats become the primary source of energy for the body, once transformed into ketone bodies, they feed the brain, and provide energy to the muscles. Suitable foods in this diet are, including butter, cream, mayonnaise, coconut oil, olive oil, avocado oil. Carbohydrates, especially in bread and starchy foods, are eliminated.

Characteristics of the ketogenic diet:

- It has a very high lipid consumption (75% of intakes)
- Intake of protein remain unchanged
- Low intake of carbohydrates
- It might cause some unpleasant symptoms in the first weeks
- Rapid weight loss
- Increase in energy
- Protection against some certain pathologies

Ketogenic diet was used to reduce seizures in children with epilepsy and it was developed in the early 1920s. It first demonstrated anticonvulsant effects in epileptic patients. In recent years, ketogenic diet has gained popularity as a fast method of losing weight. It is used to improve the symptoms of cardiovascular diseases and type 2 diabetes.

How does a ketogenic diet work?

Losing weight with ketogenic diet is characterised by the consumption of:

- 50g of carbohydrates daily which represent about 5% of the total calories which is consumed during the day.
- Lipids (75%)
- Protein (20%)

How long does the ketogenic diet last?

Ketogenic diet which is specific to weight loss has no time limit. When the ketogenic diet is practiced in the therapeutic field, it has a variable duration from a few weeks to several years depending on the expected results.

Foods that are allowed in ketogenic diet

These foods are allowed in significant quantities which are:

- Pisces
- Sea foods
- Meats
- Poultry eggs
- Butter
- Vegetal oils
- Vinegar
- Lemon juice
- olives
- Lawyer
- Vegetables that are low in carbohydrates (spinach, lettuce, kale, etc.)
- Hard cheese (100 g per day)

Here are authorized foods, but are to be consumed with moderately:

- A Whole milk
- A Whole milk yogurts
- Vegetables that are higher in carbohydrates (except carrots, beets, sweet potatoes, peas and corn)
- Wines
- Strong alcohol
- Coffee without sugar

It is very important to worry about the type of fat we eat because we ingest it a lot every day. There should be a limit to the intake of omega-6 fatty acids which is in excess and have a pro-inflammatory effect. The main sources are corn, safflower, soybean, sunflower, grape seed and wheat germ oils. It is therefore necessary to limit the consumption of vinaigrette, salad dressings and mayonnaise made from omega-6. It is advisable to consume saturated fats such as cuts of fatty meat, high-fat dairy products and monounsaturated fats such as olive oil, avocado, and nuts.

Ketogenic Diet Prohibited Foods

Ketogenic diet is very restrictive. Several foods are prohibited because they prevent the body from remaining in ketosis.

- Sugar
- Sweet products
- Cereals
- Bread
- biscuits
- legumes
- Fruits (except berries)
- Potato
- Sweet vegetables (beets, corn, carrots, etc.)
- Soft-paste cheese
- cream cheese
- Soft drinks
- Chocolate
- Honey, jams, syrup
- Juices and vegetables
- Sweet sauces
- Milk or yoghurt made from vegetable milks (soya, almonds, etc.)
- Flavoured yogurts
- Sweet fruit compotes

Advantages of the ketogenic diet

Once adapted to ketosis, it becomes rarer that one feels hunger. Indeed, the hunger-cutting side of this diet is very important. It becomes slimming to the extent that it is easier to resist the temptation of snacking.

The weight loss is often fast with this diet because they are the reserves in depths that are most used for the proper functioning of the body.

- Positive points of the ketogenic diet
- Feeling of satiety
- No caloric restriction
- Good intake of quality lipids and proteins
- Fast weight loss
- Potentially positive effect on blood lipid levels

Disadvantages of the ketogenic diet

Despite the benefits it can have, the ketogenic diet is not perfect. Indeed, it has several side effects that should not be neglected at the risk of damaging your health. You can count on the fact that:

- A Keto is too brutal with the organisations: Since the body is trained to draw its energy in the lipids, its mode of operation is more or less turned upside down. There may be nausea, severe hypoglycaemia, dehydration, cases of urinary lithiasis and a state of severe fatigue. The lack of fibre in the diet can also destabilize the digestive system.
- Promotes cardiovascular diseases: Still because of the many lipids that constitute the ketogenic diet but also the lack of fibre and other nutrients, it can sometimes develop cardiovascular disorders. This is mostly seen when the plan is followed in the long run. It may happen that those who follow the ketogenic diet suffer from atherosclerosis.
- Restricted menus: Just to see which foods are allowed and which ones to avoid, it is clear that the ketogenic diet is impractical. Over time, it can get boring and can make it difficult to go to a restaurant for example.
- Recovery of lost kilos: Like most restrictive diets, the ketogenic diet often causes a yo-yo effect. From the moment you resume a

normal diet with the presence of carbohydrates, it often happens that the lost pounds come back. The slimming effect is therefore not long term for this diet.

Why is the ketogenic diet good?

Ketogenic diet which is referred to as keto diet is low in carbohydrates and high in protein. The main goal is to gain more calories from fats and protein than carbohydrates. This works by reducing the body's sugar supply, so it can begin to break down fats and proteins into energy, thereby causing weight loss.

1. ***Help with weight loss***: It takes more work to turn fat into energy than to turn carbohydrates into energy. For this reason, a keto diet can help in speeding up weight loss. Since keto diet is high in protein, it doesn't make you hungry like other diets.

2. ***Reduces acne***: Acne can have different causes, one of which can be related to diet and blood sugar. A diet rich in refined and refined carbohydrates can alter intestinal bacteria and cause greater fluctuations in blood glucose levels, both of which can affect the health of the skin. Therefore, by decreasing the carbohydrate intake, Keto Boost Slim is not surprising that a ketogenic diet can reduce some cases of acne.

3. ***Can help reduce the risk of cancer***: The ketogenic diet has recently been the subject of much research to see how it could help prevent or even treat certain cancers. One study showed that the ketogenic diet could be an appropriate complementary treatment to chemotherapy and radiation therapy in people with cancer.

4. ***Improves heart health***: When the ketogenic diet is followed in a healthy way (which considers avocados as a healthy fat instead of pork rind), there is evidence that keto diet improves heart health by lowering the level of cholesterol.

5. ***Can protect brain function***: These can help treat or prevent diseases such as Parkinson's disease, Alzheimer's disease and even some sleep disorders. One study even found that children on the ketogenic diet had better alertness and improved cognitive functioning.

6. **Potentially reduces crises**: It is thought that the combination of proteins, carbohydrates and fats can alter the way the body uses energy, thereby resulting in ketosis.

7. ***Acidosis*** can reduce seizures in people with epilepsy. The jury has still not evaluated its effectiveness, although this seems to be more effective for children with focal seizures.

8. ***Improves health in women with PCOS***: Polycystic ovary syndrome (PCOS) is an endocrine disorder that causes ovarian hypertrophy with cysts. A high carbohydrate diet can negatively affect people with PCOS.

A week of the menu of the Ketogenic diet for men at 40

Even knowing the many foods to choose from and avoid, it is sometimes difficult to compose a menu for this type of diet. To help you in this process, here is an example of a menu for a ketogenic diet week.

DAY 1: Lunch will consist of an artichoke salad of about 75g with some sardines and olive oil. You can accompany it with a gratin to the Italian for example. As for dinner, it will have to contain a cheese soufflé consisting of a whole egg and a little cream. It is also possible to add asparagus of 25g with olive oil.

DAY 2: Endive salad with walnuts and 75g roquefort cheese and an almond and curry soup can be served for lunch. While at dinner, there will be 75g salad tomatoes and a pork chop seared with rapeseed oil.

DAY 3: To change a little, we can eat a chicken salad with coconut vinaigrette sauce and a lemon cream for dessert at lunch. In the evening, we can eat 2 cucumbers, with fresh cream and a chicken fillet.

DAY 4: For lunch, there will be 25g of grated carrots seasoned with walnut oil and accompanied by a gratin of prawns. The recipe requires 150g of prawns, a little cream and 25g of grated cheese. At dinner, the menu will be made of cauliflower florets with 1 spoon of mayonnaise. In addition to this, there will be 2 eggs in a casserole and a yoghurt.

DAY 5: The lunch menu consists of 50g of tuna tartar in addition to 25g of county. For the evening, it is advisable to eat 25g of camembert, some slices of dry sausage and 75g of mushroom with cream.

DAY 6: Roasted chicken leg with 25g of green beans and a knob of butter can make for lunch. It can even be complemented with a vanilla panna cotta and currants of 30g. At dinner, it will be an avocado with a rapeseed oil and lemon juice, and 100g of salmon marinated with olive oil and lemon.

DAY 7: At noon it is possible to eat fried lamb chop with vegetable curry (zucchini, broccoli and cauliflower). A chocolate dessert with more than 85% cocoa can complete the menu. In the evening, it is advisable to eat 100g of salmon with olive oil and lemon as well as candied tomatoes of 75g accompanied by mozzarella.

CHAPTER 6

RECIPES

To succeed in entering ketosis, it is important to compose ketogenic menus, and therefore to know the authorized foods of the keto diet. To give you more information, here are examples of good ketogenic diet recipes.

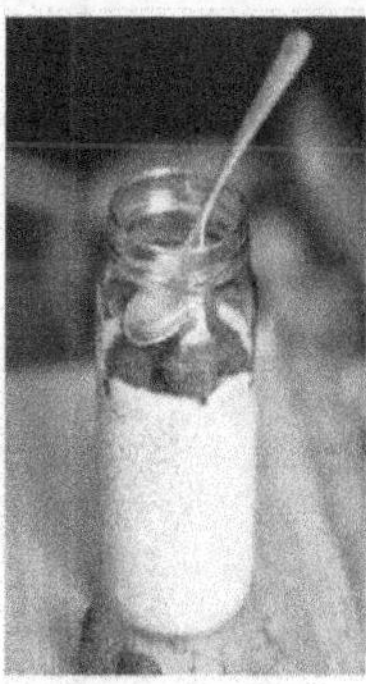

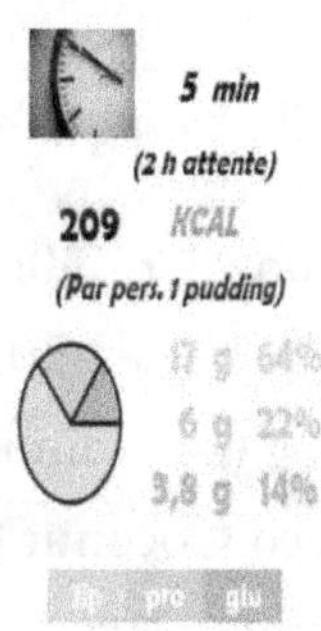

Ingredients (for 2 servings)

- Unsweetened Coconut Milk - 120g
- Chia Seeds - 40g
- Frozen Raspberries - 60g
- Erythritol / Stevia - 10g

Preparation

- Mix the coconut milk and chia seeds. Flavor with cinnamon, a few drops of vanilla extract or orange blossom
- Reserve in the fridge for 2 hours
- Meanwhile defrost raspberries
- Add raspberries over pudding, sprinkle with stevia / erythritol type sweetener if needed and enjoy

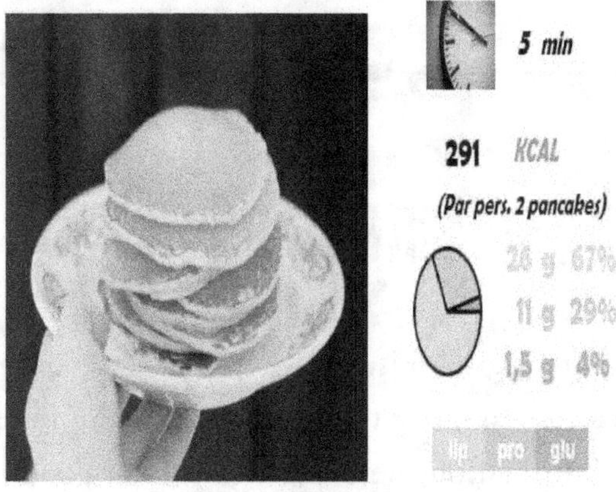

Pancake keto

Ingredients (for 2 servings - 4 pancakes)

- Almond powder - 30g
- Whipped Cheese - 30g
- Egg - 106g (4 medium eggs)
- Deodorized Coconut Oil - 10g
- Sweet Butter - 10g

Preparation

- Heat the coconut oil in the microwave
- In another bowl beat the eggs and add the whipped cheese and almond powder
- Heat a pan with a knob of sweet butterServe salted with a fried fresh egg or sweetened with sugar free syrup type Frankys

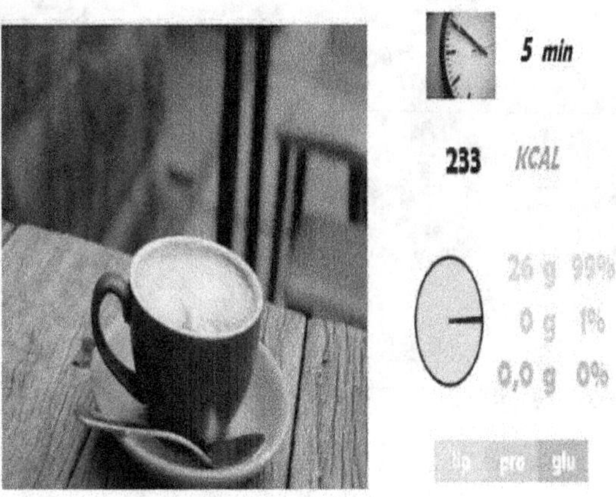

Bulletproof Coffee

Ingredients

- Black Coffee - 200g
- Coconut Oil - 10g
- Sweet Butter - 20g

Preparation

- Pour a big black coffee
- In a shaker, mix the coffee with the butter (or the whole cream) and coconut oil.
- If necessary, sweetened with stevia sweetener or erythritol

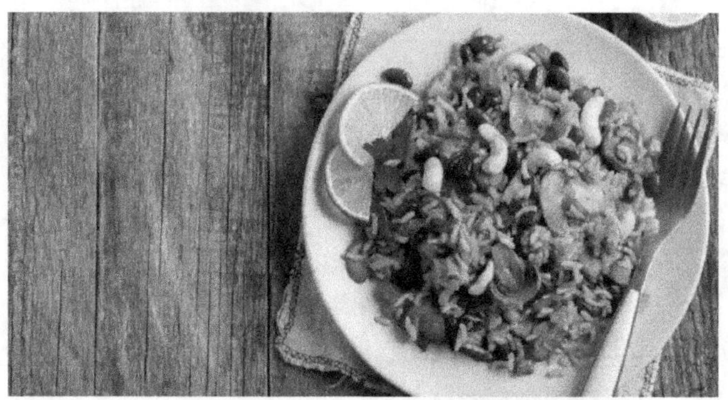

Fried Rice with Red Beans, Cashews and Peppers

Ingredients

- 400g cooked rice
- 1 red pepper
- 150g cooked red beans
- 150g of cashew nuts
- 3 tablespoons of olive oil
- 1g of gomasio

Preparation

- Wash and seed red pepper, then cut into small pieces.
- Heat the oil in a skillet. Pour the rice and brown it.
- Add pepper pieces, well-drained beans and cashews. Stir and heat uncovered for a few minutes.
- Sprinkle with flour, stir and serve hot.

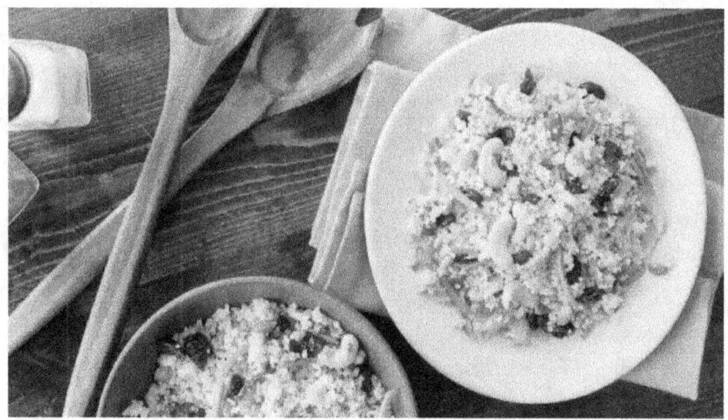

Tabbouleh with Carrots, Cranberries and Cashews

Ingredients

- 200g of wheat semolina
- 3 carrots
- 100g unsalted cashews
- 50g of squash seeds
- 3 tablespoons walnut oil
- 1 lemon
- 1 tablespoon of chopped fresh coriander
- Salt & Pepper

Preparation

- In a salad bowl, put the semolina and cover with water.
- Squeeze the lemon over, salt, pepper and mix. Allow to swell about twenty minutes stirring regularly with a fork.
- Meanwhile, let the dried cranberries swell in a little water.
- Peel the carrots and grate them not too finely.
- Mix grated carrots, drained cranberries, cashews and pumpkin seeds with couscous.
- Sprinkle with walnut oil, sprinkle with coriander and mix.
- Put it in the fridge.

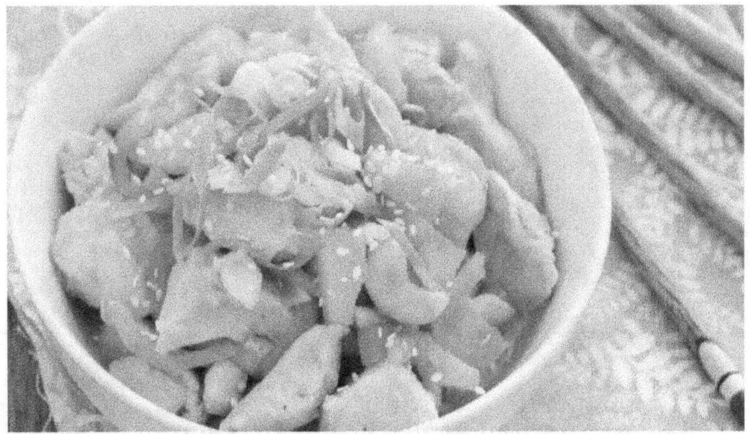

Slimming Chicken with Cashew Nuts and Pineapple

Ingredients

- 2 tablespoons grated coconut
- 80 g raw cashews
- 2 tablespoons sunflower oil
- 1 onion, peeled and cut into pieces
- 4 cloves garlic, peeled and thinly sliced
- 350 g chicken breast cut into pieces
- ½ green pepper seeded and cut into strips
- ½ red pepper seeded and sliced
- 320 g pineapple
- 3 onions cleaned and chopped
- 2 tablespoons oyster sauce
- 1 tablespoon fish sauce
- 1 teaspoon of sugar
- 2 teaspoons red pepper powder

Preparation

- Preheat the oven to 180 ° C.
- Then spread the coconut on a baking sheet which is lined with parchment paper.

- Then grill in the hot oven for about 10 minutes.
- Stir occasionally.
- Remove it from the oven and then reserve it.
- Spread the cashews over the baking sheet and grill for 15 minutes until golden brown. Remove from the oven and let cool.
- You have to heat the oil in a large skillet on medium heat.
- Then add the garlic, onion and chilli.
- Remove from the pan and increase the heat. This time, saute the chicken and peppers twice, until the chicken is light brown. Put the onion / chilli mixture back in the pan, add the oyster sauce, fish sauce, sugar and pineapple in pieces and cook for 2 minutes, stirring occasionally.
- Add the coconut, roasted cashews and onions to the chicken mixture and mix.
- Savor without delay.

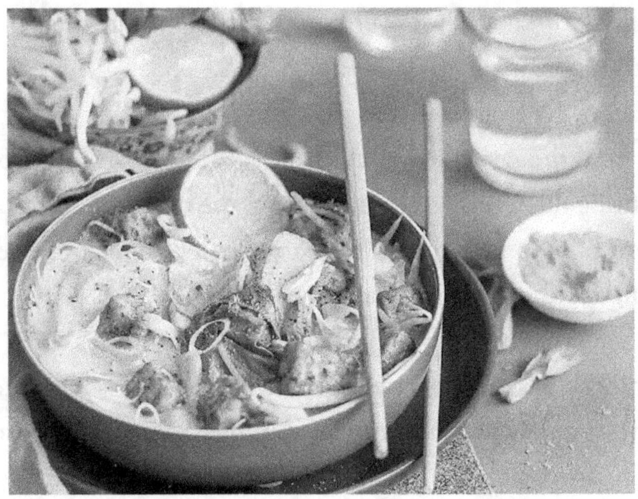

Asian Vegetable and Tempeh Soup

This recipe is vegetarian and ketogenic. The rice vermicelli from the original recipe is replaced here with konjac pasta that is free of carbohydrates.

Ingredients

- 2 cups of vegetables soup 500 mL
- 1 cup of water 250 mL
- ⅓ cup unsweetened coconut milk 85 mL
- ½ limes / limes, juice and zest 35 g
- 1 little bok choy 150 g
- ½ dried red peppers, finely chopped 0.2 g
- 200 g shirataki noodles / konjac
- 4 teaspoons coconut oil 18 g
- 240 g tempeh, cut into cubes
- 1 teaspoon   curry / curry powder   3 g
- 1 pinch salt [optional] 0.2 g
- pepper to taste [optional]
- ½ carrots, finely grated 50 g
- ½ green onions / shallots, chopped
- 9 tablespoons bean sprouts 40 g

- Rinse the noodles with plenty of water to eliminate the odor and drain well.
- In a saucepan, bring broth, water, coconut milk, zest and lime juice to a boil.
- Add the bok choy and red pepper.
- Reserve on a low heat.
- Meanwhile, heat a skillet over medium heat. Add noodles and cook for 2-3 minutes, stirring until all the noodles are hot.
- Then move the noodles from the pan and set it aside.
- Heat the oil over medium-high heat in the skillet.
- Cook until golden brown, about 5 min.
- Salt and pepper.
- Prepare the vegetables by grating the carrots and slicing the green onions.
- Spread in the bowls with the sprouts, noodles, tempeh cubes and cooking oil. Pour broth over.
- Serve.

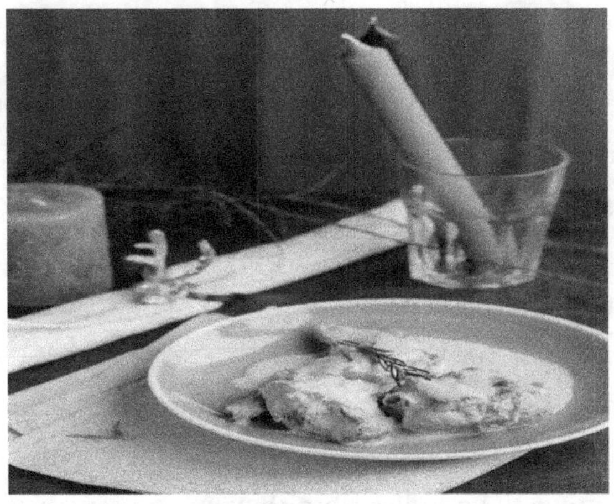

Creamy Rabbit with Mustard

Rabbit meat is white, a little similar to chicken in taste and texture. It is found more and more commonly in supermarkets, because the rabbit combines a fine and delicate taste with very interesting nutritional qualities. Indeed it is a meat rich in proteins, vitamins and minerals, and at the same time low fat and very digestible. Serve it with a classic ketogenic diet: cauliflower rice.

Ingredients

- 1 rabbit, cut into 6-8 pieces 1.4 kg
- 2 tablespoons olive oil 30 mL
- 1 pinch salt [optional] 0.2 g
- pepper to taste [optional]
- 1 onion, finely chopped 200 g
- 2 pods garlic, finely chopped
- ½ cup White wine 125 mL
- 1 cup   chicken broth 250 mL
- 2 bay leaves 0.4 g
- ¼ cup whipping cream 35% 65 mL
- 3 tablespoons whole grain mustard

- Before you start, heat the oven to 175 ° C / 350 ° F.
- In a casserole, cover the rabbit in oil over medium-high heat.
- Salt and pepper.
- Reserve the rabbit on a plate. Add onion and garlic and cook until softened, about 3 minutes.
- Add the wine and scrape the bottom thoroughly. Put the rabbit back in the casserole. Add broth and bring to boil. Add the bay leaf. Mix well.
- Cover and bake for 2 hours, until meat is easily flaked with a fork.
- Meanwhile, in a small bowl, mix the cream and mustard.
- Remove the casserole from the oven. Remove the rabbit, bone it and reserve the meat. Using a whisk, add the cream mixture to the cooking juices in the casserole.
- Heat 2-3 min on the stove.
- Return the rabbit meat to the casserole to warm and serve.

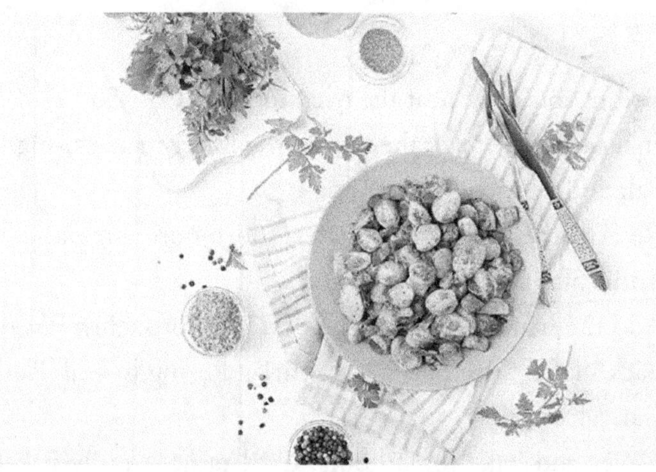

Brussel Sprouts Braised with Bacon

Green vegetables have their place on the ketogenic menu. In this recipe, Brussels sprouts become tender with a small smoky taste. Delicious!

Ingredients

- 2 slices bacon, chopped 40 g
- 2 tablespoons olive oil 30 mL
- 14 Brussels sprouts, cut in half or in four 360 g
- 1 cup chicken broth 250 mL
- 2 teaspoons whole grain mustard 10 g
- 1 pinch salt [optional] 0.2 g
- pepper to taste [optional]

Preparation

- Chop the bacon and place it in a non-stick pan. Fry until crisp, then set aside on a sheet of paper.
- Add oil and meat at medium heat.
- Put cabbage and cook for 2 minutes while stirring.
- Add broth and mustard, cover, and simmer until cabbage is tender, about 7 min. Discover, and continue to simmer until the liquid is evaporated, about 7 min.

- Put the bacon back in the skillet.
- Cook 1 min stirring.
- Salt and pepper.
- Serve.

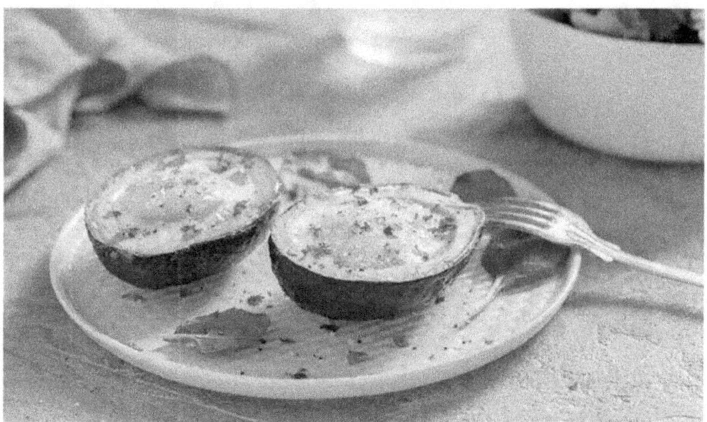

Cauliflower Popcorn

Ingredients

- Parchment paper
- ⅓ cup olive oil 85 mL
- ¼ cup wine vinegar 65 mL
- ¼ teaspoon paprika 0.4 g
- 1 pinch cayenne pepper 0.1 g
- ⅛ teaspoons salt [optional] 0.4 g
- 6 cups cauliflower, cut into bunches of uniform size 1 kg

Preparation

- Before you start, heat the oven to 230 ° C / 450°F. Line a large baking sheet with parchment paper.
- Pour the oil, vinegar, spices and salt into a large bowl. Mix everything well.
- Cut the cauliflower into small bouquets of uniform size, then put in the bowl with the vinaigrette. Toupin everything to coat

vinaigrette bouquets. Spread these on the plate.

- Bake in the center of the oven until cauliflower is golden and tender but crisp, about 25-30 min.
- Serve hot or at room temperature.

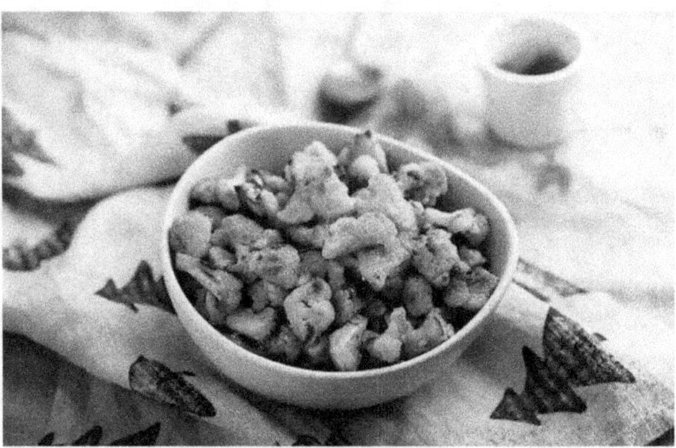

Avocado Egg Casserole

This recipe is very easy to make. Its presentation is cool and perfect for brunch or a light meal.

Ingredients

- Aluminium foil
- 2 lawyers 340 g
- 4 big calibre eggs
- 1 pinch salt [optional] 0.2 g
- Pepper to taste [optional]
- 1 pinch Cayenne pepper 0.1 g
- 2 teaspoons fresh chives, finely chopped [optional] 2 g

Preparation

- Before you start, heat the oven to 220 ° C / 425 ° F. Cover the baking sheet with foil.
- Slice the avocados in half
- Then remove the core.

- Using a spoon, remove about a spoonful or more of avocado flesh to create a hollow large enough to deposit an egg.
- Put the avocados on the plate and fold the foil around the avocados to prevent them from tipping over. Alternatively put each lawyer in a ramekin.
- Break one egg into each avocado half taking care not to break the yolk. Add salt and pepper to taste. Add a pinch of Cayenne.
- Place it at the center of the oven, then bake for 15-18 min. Or until the whites have seared and the yolks are still a little runny.
- Garnish with chopped chives and serve.

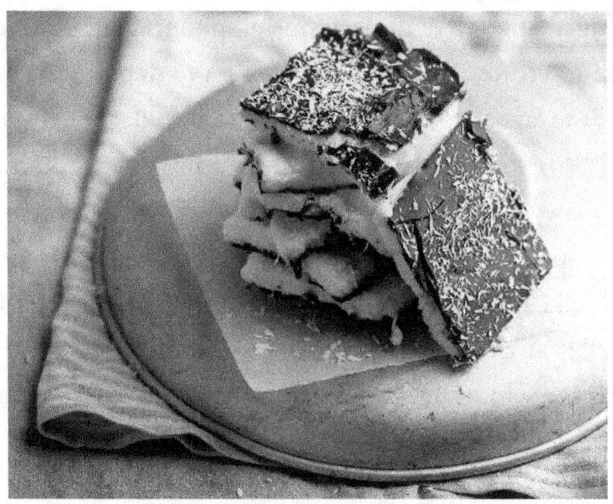

"Fat bombs" Cheesecake

Fat bombs are used to meet lipid needs. For the sweet side, a small amount of stevia is used instead of sugar.

Ingredients

- parchment paper
- 3 ½ tablespoons unsalted butter 50 g
- 4 tablespoons coconut oil 55 g
- 1 cup cream cheese 150 g
- 8 drops liquid stevia [optional] 0.63 mL
- ½ lemons, for juice and zest 60 g
- 1 tablespoon grated coconut (in filaments), unsweetened 5 g
- 1 teaspoon coconut oil, for chocolate 5 g
- 50 g bitter chocolate (black)

Preparation

- Prepare 12 small silicone molds or line up a 20x20 cm (8x8 ") square parchment paper pan to facilitate demolding.
- Melt the butter and coconut oil in the microwave in 15 sec intervals. Add cream cheese and mix well. Add drops of stevia

(optional), the juice and zest of lemon and the grated coconut, mix. Spread the mixture in the mold.

- Melt chocolate with coconut oil in the microwave at 15-second intervals.
- Spread on the cream cheese mixture.
- Refrigerate until solid, about 1 hr.
- Unmould on a work surface and remove the paper. Cut into squares, to get 12 pieces.

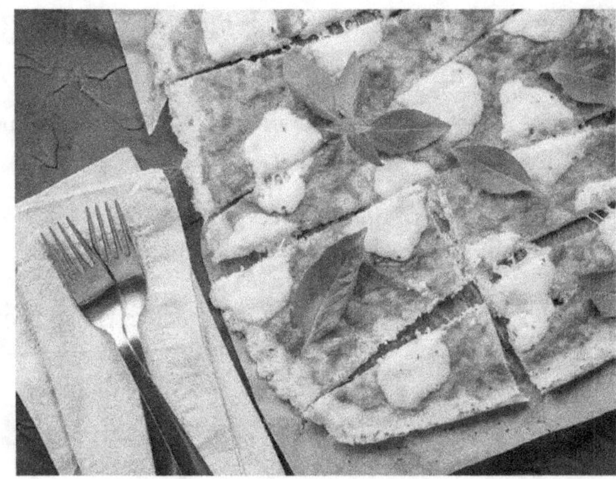

Cheese and Tomato Pizza With Cauliflower Crust

Fat bombs are used to meet lipid needs. For the sweet side, a small amount of stevia is used instead of sugar.

Ingredients

- 3 cups cauliflower 500 g
- 1 clove garlic, minced
- 2 big caliber eggs
- ⅛ teaspoons salt 0.4 g
- ¼ cup of Mother's tomato sausage 65 mL
- 4 anchovy fillets 16 g
- 2 bocconcini / mozzarella 110 g
- Pepper to taste [optional]
- 8 leaves fresh basil 4 g

Preparation

- Before you start, heat the oven to 205 ° C / 400° F. Line a large baking sheet with parchment paper.
- Prepare the cauliflower and cut into bouquets and transfer to the cup of a food processor. Operate until the cauliflower is finely chopped. Transfer to a large bowl.

- Add eggs, salt and minced garlic. Mix well and spread the mixture over the pizza crust.
- Bake in the center of the oven until golden, about 20 minutes.
- Remove the baking sheet from the oven.
- Then add the tomato sauce, anchovies and cheese to the crust.
- Put the plate back in the oven for 10-15 min. Garnish with basil leaves and serve.

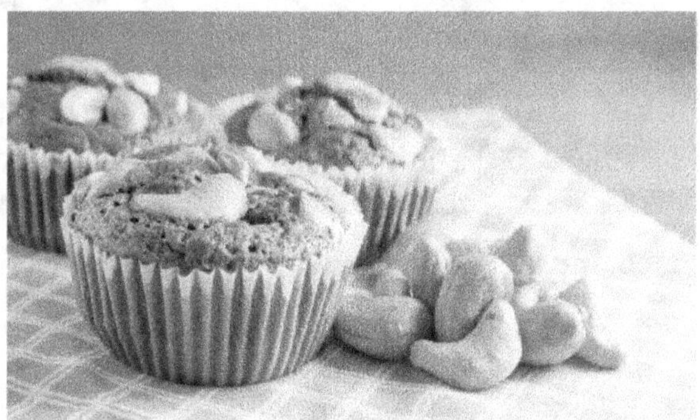

Chocolate and Cashew Nut Slimming Mini Cakes

Ingredients

- 3 eggs
- 150g of dark chocolate
- 100g of sugar
- 100g of cashew nuts
- 70g of flour

Preparation

- Preheat the oven to 200 ° C (th.6-7).
- Melt chocolate in a bain-marie or microwave.
- Mix the cashews finely.
- In a salad bowl, mix the eggs with the sugar, flour, cashew powder, then pour the melted chocolate and mix well until a smooth paste.
- Pour the dough into small cake molds.
- Bake for around 20 minutes.

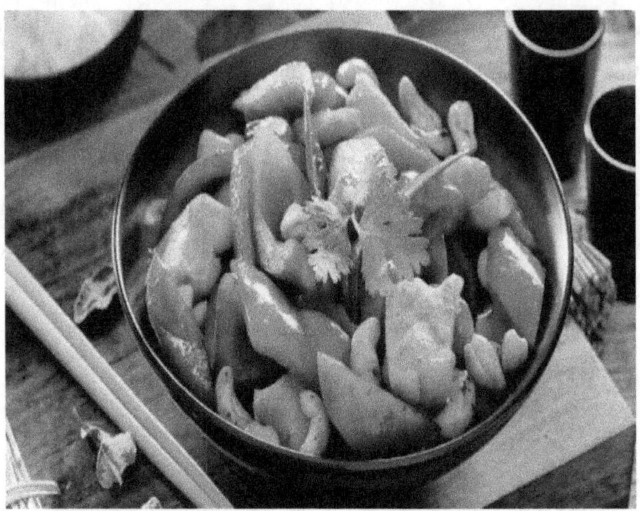

Spinach and Red Kidney Bean With Cashew Nuts

Ingredients

- 200g chopped spinach
- 150g cooked red beans
- 150g of cashew nuts
- 3 eggs
- 40cl of light cream
- Salt & Pepper

Preparation

- Preheat the oven to (180 °).
- Whisk the eggs with the sieve corn, cream, paprika, salt and pepper in a bowl.
- Roughly chop the cashews and mix them with the mixture.
- In a gratin dish, place the spinach and kidney beans well drained, then pour the mixture on it.
- Bake for about 25 minutes.

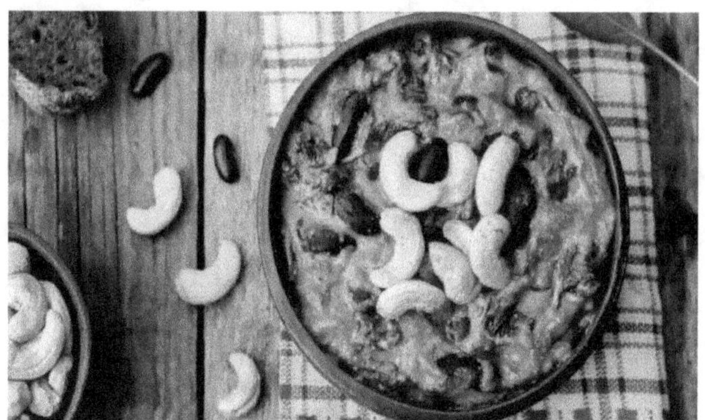

Chicken Wok with Gourmet Peas, Peppers and Cashew Nuts

Ingredients

- 4 chicken breasts
- 2 green peppers
- 1 red pepper
- 100g of gourmet peas
- 1 big onion
- ½ red pepper
- 75g of cashew nuts
- Olive oil
- Salt & Pepper

Preparation

- Peel and finely slice the onion.
- Wash, seed and cut peppers into pieces.
- Tease the greedy peas.
- Cut the chicken into pieces.
- Wash, seed and chop the chili into small pieces.
- Heat olive oil in a skillet and cook the onion, chicken and chilli until the chicken is golden brown.
- Add the sweet peas and peppers, salt and pepper.
- Add the chilli and cashews and sauté until the sweet peas and peppers are cooked.
- Serve immediately with white rice.

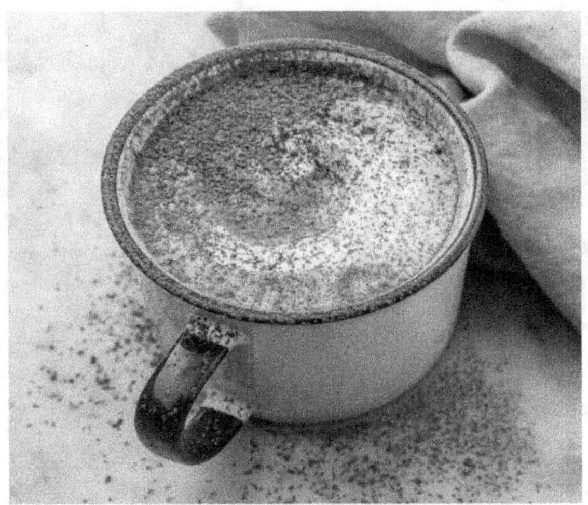

Keto Hot Chocolate

Ingredients

- 2 tbsp. unsweetened cocoa powder, plus more for garnish
- 2 ½ tsp. keto-friendly sugar, such as Swerve
- 1 ¼ c. water
- ¼ c. heavy cream
- ¼ tsp. pure vanilla extract
- Whipped cream, for serving

Preparation

- In a saucepan over medium-low heat, whisk cocoa.
- Then, mix and stir in 2 tablespoons of water or until it is smooth and dissolved.
- Increase heat to medium, add remaining water and cream, and whisk occasionally until hot.
- Stir in vanilla, then pour it into a mug.
- Serve it with whipped cream and a dusting of cocoa powder.

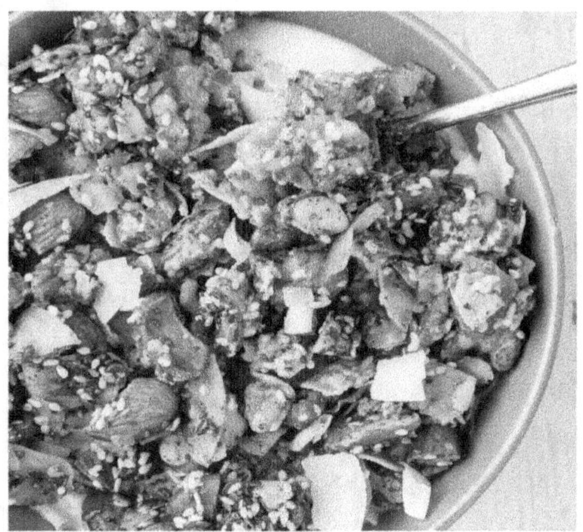

Keto Cereal

Make a big batch of this granola and have an easy breakfast ready all week long. It even goes great sprinkled on keto Ice Cream.

INGREDIENTS

- Cooking spray
- 1 c. almonds, chopped
- 1 c. walnuts, chopped
- 1 c. unsweetened coconut flakes
- ¼ c. sesame seeds
- 2 tbsp. flax seeds
- 2 tbsp. chia seeds
- ½ tsp. ground clove
- 1 ½ tsp. ground cinnamon
- 1 tsp. pure vanilla extract
- ½ tsp. kosher salt
- 1 large egg white
- ¼ c. melted coconut oil

- Firstly, preheat the oven to 350°.
- Then grease a baking sheet with cooking spray.
- Mix walnuts, almond, sesame seeds, coconut flakes, flax seeds and chia seeds together in a large bowl.
- Then stir with cinnamon, vanilla, salt and cloves.
- Then beat egg white until it becomes foamy.
- Stir with granola.
- Then add coconut oil.
- Stir it until everything becomes well coated.
- Then pour everything into the prepared baking sheet and spread them into an oven layer.
- Bake it for 20 to 25 minutes, or until it is golden.
- Then gently stir halfway through.
- Let cool completely.

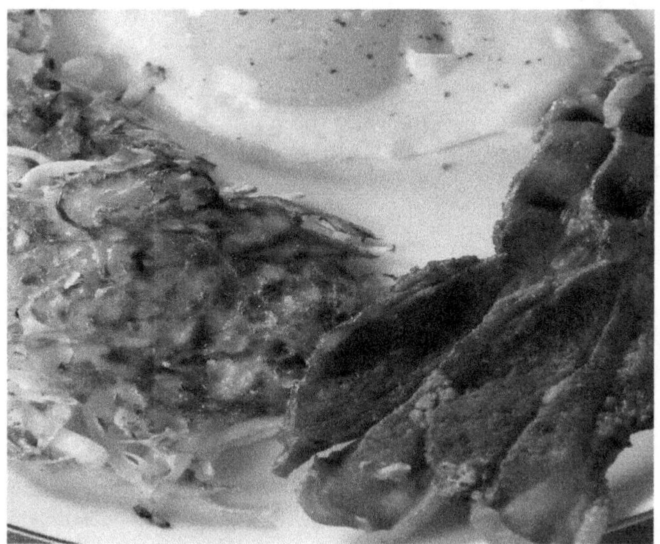

Cabbage Hash Browns

Ingredients

- 2 large eggs
- ½ tsp. garlic powder
- ½ tsp. kosher salt
- Freshly ground black pepper
- 2 c. shredded cabbage
- ¼ small yellow onion, thinly sliced
- 1 tbsp. vegetable oil

Preparations

- Whisk garlic powder, salt and eggs in a large bowl.
- Then add black pepper seasoning.
- Add two eggs (whisk) ,onion and cabbage then toss to combine.
- Heat the oil in a large skillet.
- Then divide the mixture into four patties on the pan, press with spatula to flatten
- Cook for about 3 minutes per side.

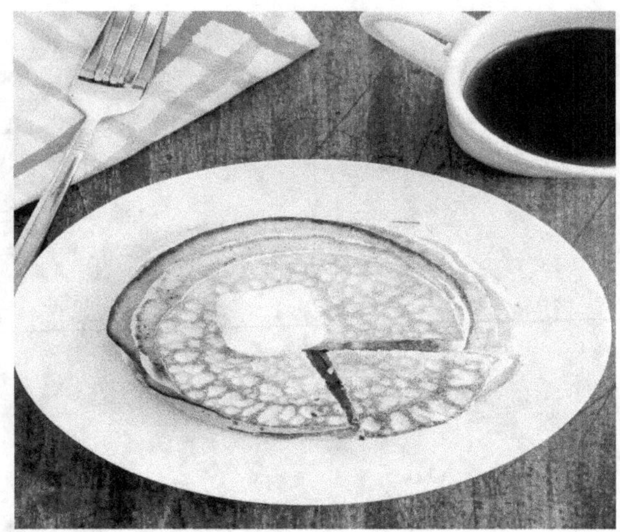

Pancakes

Ingredients

- ½ c. almond flour
- 4 oz. cream cheese, softened
- 4 large eggs
- 1 tsp. lemon zest
- Butter, for frying and serving

Preparations

- Whisk cream cheese, eggs, lemon zest, and almond flour in a medium bowl until it becomes smooth.
- Melt 1 tablespoon butter.
- Pour 3 tablespoons batter and cook it for about 2 minutes. Then flip it and cook it for about 2 minutes
- Transfer it to a plate, then continue with the rest of the batter.
- Serve it with butter on top.

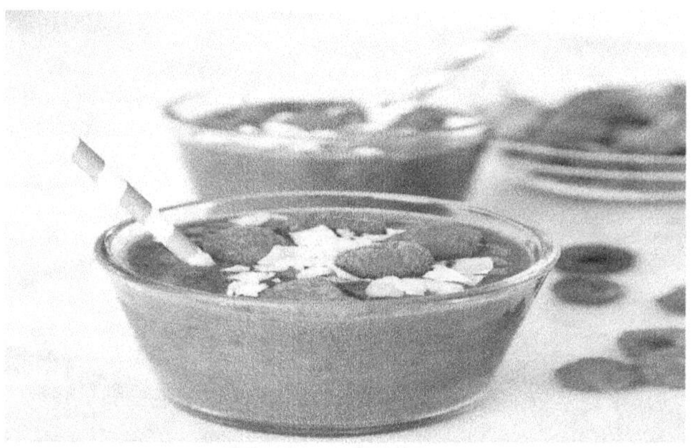

Keto Smoothie

There are smoothies that are lower in carbs like Raspberry, blackberry, strawberry. They are lower in carbs than other smoothie fruits like bananas, pineapples, and mangoes.

Ingredients

- 1 ½ c. frozen strawberries
- 1 ½ c. frozen raspberries, plus more for garnish (optional)
- 1 c. frozen blackberries
- 2 c. coconut milk
- 1 c. baby spinach
- Unsweetened shaved coconut, for garnish (optional)

Preparation

- Blend all the ingredients using a blender except coconut.
- Blend it until it becomes very smooth.
- Serve with raspberries and coconut on top.

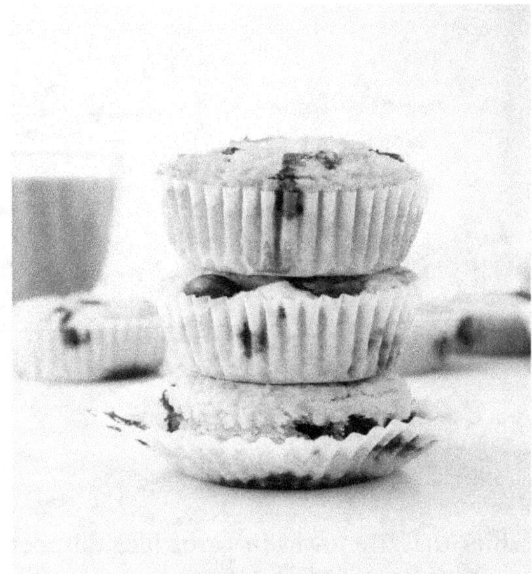

Keto Breakfast Cups

Ingredients

- 2 lb. ground pork
- 1 tbsp. freshly chopped thyme
- 2 cloves garlic, minced
- ½ tsp. paprika
- ½ tsp. ground cumin
- 1 tsp. kosher salt
- Freshly ground black pepper
- 2 ½ c. chopped fresh spinach
- 1 c. shredded white cheddar
- 12 eggs
- 1 tbsp. freshly chopped chives

Preparation

- Preheat your oven at 400°C.
- Combine thyme, ground pork, paprika, garlic, salt and cumin.
- Then season with pepper.
- Then add a small handful of pork to each of the muffin tin.

- Then press the sides to create a cup.
- Divide spinach and cheese equally between cups.
- Then crack an egg on top of each cup and add salt and pepper seasoning.
- Bake the eggs until they are set and the sausage is done for about 25 minutes.
- Garnish with chives
- Then serve.

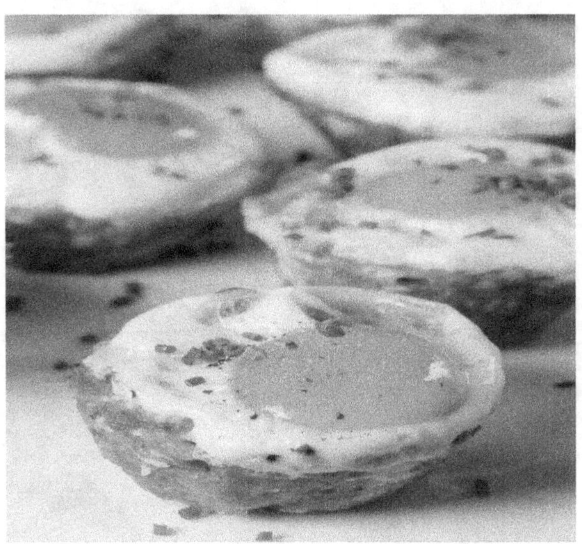

Keto Blueberry Muffins

Ingredients

- 2 ½ c. almond flour
- 1 ⅓ c. keto friendly sugar (such as Swerve)
- 1 ½ tsp. baking powder
- ½ tsp. baking soda
- ½ tsp. kosher salt
- ⅓ c. melted butter
- ⅓ c. unsweetened almond milk
- 3 large eggs
- 1 tsp. pure vanilla extract
- ⅔ c. fresh blueberries
- Zest of ½ lemon (optional)

Preparation

- Preheat the oven to about 350°C.
- Then line a 12-cup muffin pan with cupcake liners.
- Combine and whisk almond flour, baking powder, baking soda, and salt.

- Whisk in melted butter, almond milk, eggs, and vanilla until just combined.
- Gently fold blueberries and lemon zest (if using) until evenly distributed. Scoop equal amounts of batter into each cupcake liner and bake until slightly golden and a toothpick inserted into the center of a muffin comes out clean, 23 minutes. Let cool slightly before serving.

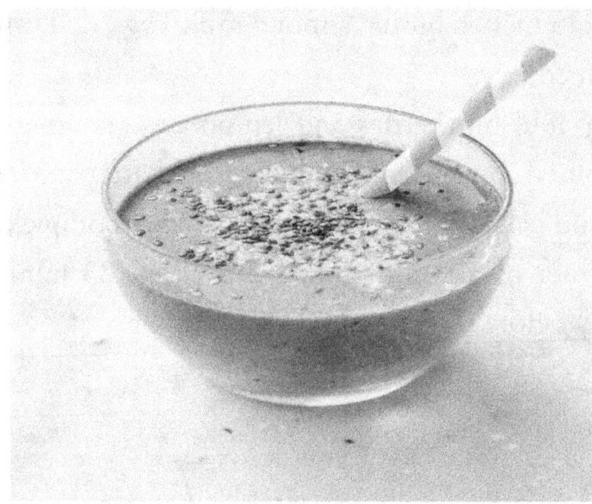

Chocolate Keto Protein Shake

Who needs protein powder anyways? Packed with almond milk, almond butter, chia seeds, and hemp seeds, this shake will energize you and keep you full all morning. If you're not really a chocolate person and prefer fruit smoothies, Coconut Berry Keto Smoothie is for you.

Ingredients

- ¾ c. almond milk
- ½ ice
- Two tablespoon of almond butter
- Two tablespoons of unsweetened cocoa powder
- Two to three tablespoon of keto-friendly sugar substitute to taste
- One tablespoon of chia seeds.
- Two tablespoon of hemp seeds.
- ½ tablespoon of pure vanilla extract
- Pinch of kosher salt

Preparation

- Combine and blend all the ingredients until it is smooth.
- Pour it into a glass
- Garnish it with more chia and hemp seeds.

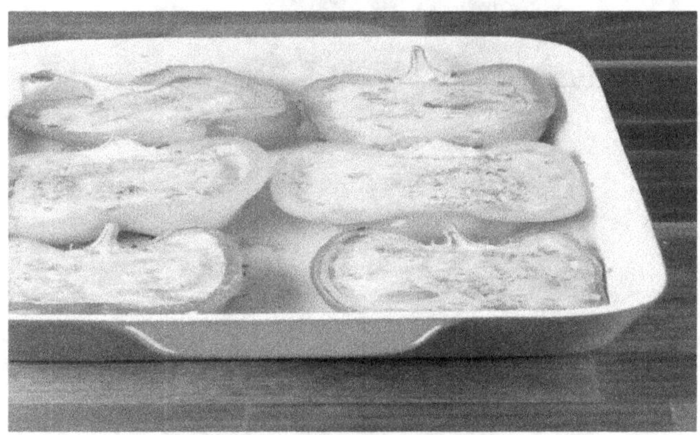

Bell *Pepper* Eggs

Ingredients

- One bell pepper, sliced ir into 1/4" rings
- Six eggs
- Kosher salt
- Freshly ground black pepper
- Two tablespoon of chopped chives
- Two tablespoon of chopped parsley

Preparation

- Heat a skillet over medium heat.
- Grease it lightly with cooking spray.
- Place a bell pepper ring in the skillet, then saute it for two minutes.
- Flip the ring, then crack an egg in the middle.
- Salt and pepper with seasoning, then cook until the egg is cooked to your liking, 2 to 4 minutes.
- Repeat with the other eggs, then garnish with chives and parsley.

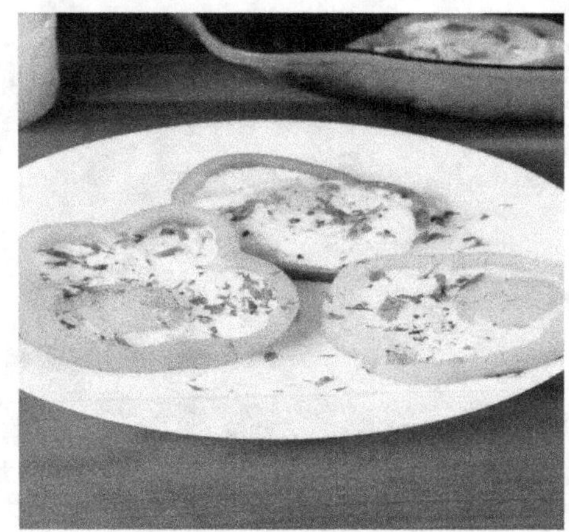

Omelet-Stuffed Peppers

Ingredients

- 2 bell peppers, halved and seeds removed
- 8 eggs, lightly beaten
- ¼ c. milk
- 4 slices bacon, cooked and crumbled
- 1 c. shredded cheddar
- 2 tbsp. finely chopped chives, plus more for garnish
- Kosher salt
- Freshly cracked black pepper

Preparation

- Preheat the oven.
- Place the pepper cut side up in a large baking dish.
- Add a little water to the dish, then bake peppers for five minutes.
- Beat milk and egg, then stir in cheese, bacon and chives.
- Add salt and pepper seasoning
- When peppers are done baking, pour egg mixture into peppers.
- Place back in the oven and bake 35 to 40 minutes more, until eggs are set.
- Garnish with more chives and serve.

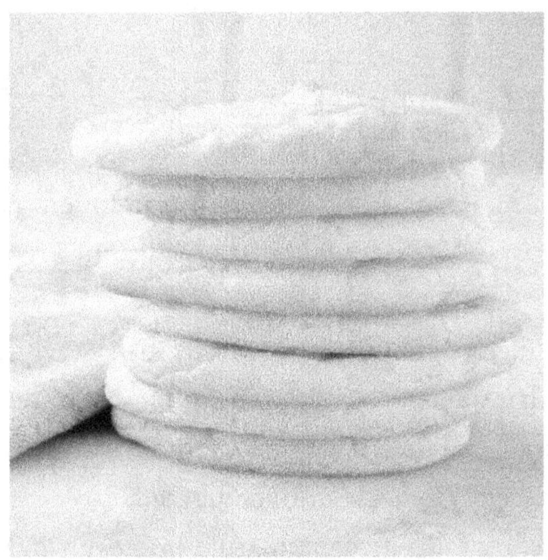

Keto Cloud Bread

Ingredients

- FOR PLAIN CLOUD BREAD
- 3 large eggs, at room temperature
- ¼ tsp. cream of tartar
- Pinch of kosher salt
- 2 oz. cream cheese, softened
- FOR PIZZA CLOUD BREAD
- 1 tbsp. Italian seasoning
- 2 tbsp. shredded mozzarella or grated Parmesan
- 2 tsp. tomato paste
- FOR EVERYTHING BAGEL CLOUD BREAD
- 1/8 tsp. kosher salt
- 1 tsp. Poppy seeds
- 1 tsp. sesame seeds
- 1 tsp. minced dried garlic
- 1 tsp. minced dried onion
- FOR RANCH CLOUD BREAD
- 1 ½ tsp. ranch seasoning powder

- PLAIN CLOUD BREAD
- Firstly, preheat the oven at 300°
- Then, line a large baking sheet with parchment paper.
- Then separate the egg whites from yolks into two medium glass bowls.
- Then add cream of tartar and salt to the egg whites.
- Using a hand mixer, beat it until stiff peaks from, 2 to 3 minutes.
- Add the cream cheese to egg yolks, then, using a hand mixer, mix yolks and cream cheese until combined.
- Then, gently fold egg yolk mixture into egg whites.
- Divide the mixture into eight mounds on a prepared baking sheet, spacing them about 4" apart.
- Then bake until golden, 25 to 30 minutes.
- Immediately sprinkle each piece of bread with cheese and bake until melty, 2 to 3 minutes more.
- Cool slightly.
- PIZZA CLOUD BREAD:
- In the egg yolk mixture, add 1 tablespoon of italian seasoning, 2 tablespoon of shredded mozzarella or grated Parmesan, and 2 teaspoons tomato paste.
- EVERYTHING BAGEL CLOUD BREAD:
- In the egg yolk mixture, add ⅛ teaspoon of kosher salt.
- 1 teaspoon of poppy seeds.
- 1 teaspoon of sesame seeds.
- 1 teaspoon of minced dried garlic
- 1 teaspoon of minced dried onion.
- RANCH CLOUD BREAD:
- In the egg yolk mixture, add 1½ teaspoons ranch seasoning powder.

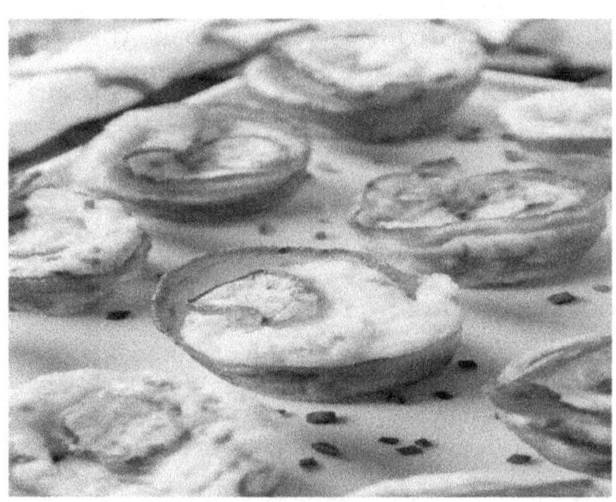

Jalapeño Popper Egg Cups

Ingredients

- 12 slices of bacon
- 10 large eggs
- ¼ sour cream
- ½ shredded Cheddar
- ½ shredded mozzarella
- 2 jalapeños, 1 minced and 1 thinly sliced
- 1 tablespoon of garlic powder
- kosher salt
- Freshly ground black pepper
- nonstick cooking spray

Preparations

- Preheat the oven at 375°.
- Cook bacon until it is slightly browned but still pliable.
- Then set aside on a paper towel-lined plate to drain.
- Whisk together eggs, sour cream, cheeses, minced jalapeño and garlic powder.
- Then season with salt and pepper.
- Use nonstick cooking spray, grease a muffin tin.

- Line each well with one slice of bacon, then pour egg mixture into each muffin cup until about two-thirds of the way to the top.
- Then top each muffin with a jalapeño slices.
- Bake it for 20 minutes, or until the eggs no longer look wet.
- Then cool slightly before removing from the muffin tin.
- Serve.

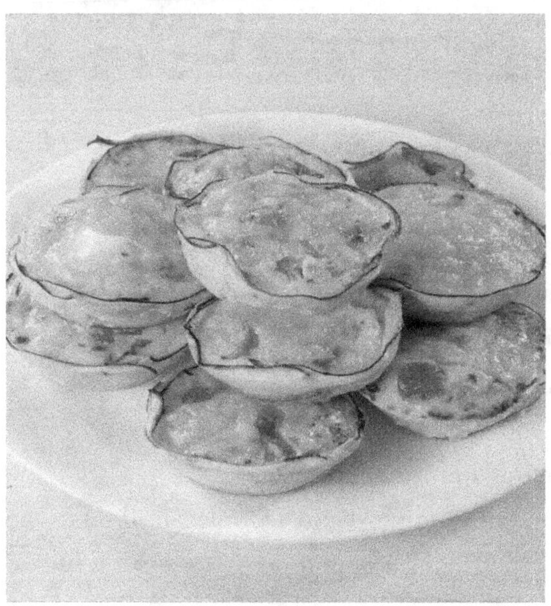

Zucchini Egg Cups

INGREDIENTS

- Cooking spray, for pan
- 2 zucchinis, peeled into strips
- ¼ lb. ham, chopped
- ½ c. cherry tomatoes, quartered
- 8 eggs
- ½ c. heavy cream
- Kosher salt
- Freshly ground black pepper

- ½ tsp. dried oregano
- 1 c. Pinch red pepper flakes
- 1 c. shredded cheddar

PREPARATIONS

- Preheat the oven at 400°.
- Then grease a muffin tin with cooking spray.
- After that, line the inside and bottom of the muffin tin with zucchini strips, to form a crust.
- Sprinkle the ham and cherry tomatoes inside each crust.
- Whisk together eggs, heavy cream, oregano, and red pepper flakes then season with salt and pepper.
- Then pour egg mixture over ham and tomatoes then top with cheese.
- Bake it until eggs are set, 30 minutes.

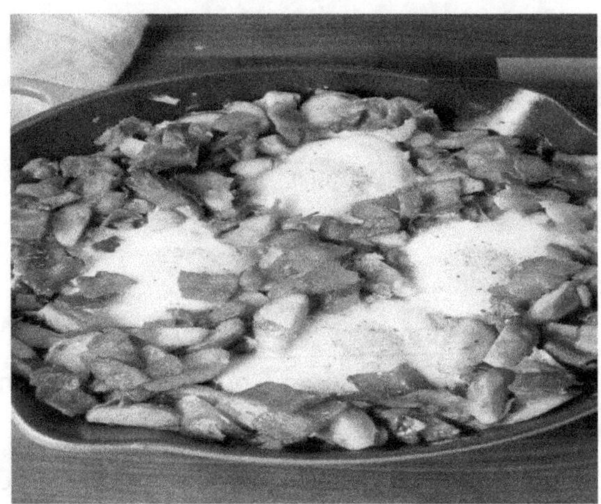

Brussels Sprouts Hash

INGREDIENTS

- 6 slices bacon, cut into 1" pieces
- ½ onion, chopped
- 1 lb. Brussels sprouts, trimmed and quartered
- Kosher salt
- Freshly ground black pepper
- ¼ tsp. crushed red pepper flakes
- 2 cloves garlic, minced
- 4 large eggs

PREPARATIONS

- Cook bacon until crispy in a large skillet over medium heat.
- Then turn off heat and transfer the bacon to a paper towel-lined plate.
- Keep most of the bacon fat in the skillet, remove any black pieces from the pan.
- Add onion and brussels sprouts to the skillet.
- Cook and keep stirring occasionally until the vegetables begin to soften and turn golden.
- Season it with salt, pepper, and red pepper flakes.

- Add two tablespoons of water and cover the skillet.
- Cook until the brussels sprouts are tender and water has evaporated for about 5 minutes. If all the water evaporates before the brussels sprouts are tender, then add more water to the skillet and cover for a couple minutes more.
- Add garlic to skillet and cook until fragrant, 1 minute.
- Using a wooden spoon, make four holes in the hash to reveal the bottom of the skillet.
- Crack the egg into each hole and season each egg with salt and pepper.
- Replace the lid and cook until eggs are cooked to your liking, about 5 minutes for a just runny egg.
- Sprinkle cooked bacon bits over the entire skillet and serve warm.

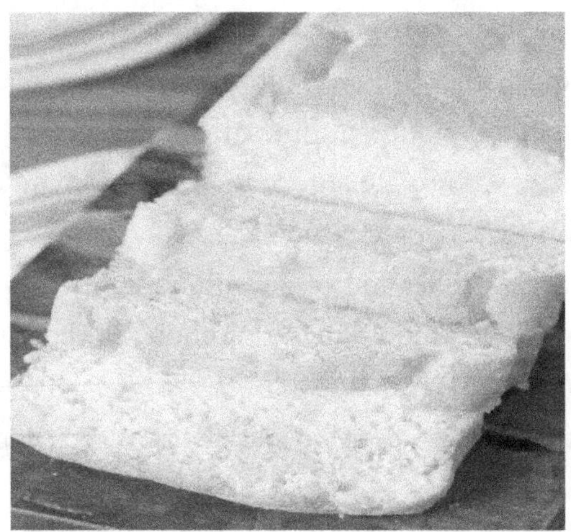

Keto Bread

INGREDIENTS

- 6 large eggs
- ½ tsp. cream of tartar
- ¼ c. (½ stick) butter, melted and cooled
- 1 ½ c. finely ground almond flour
- 1 tbsp. baking powder
- ½ tsp. kosher salt

PREPARATIONS

- Preheat the oven to about 375° and then line an 8"-x-4" loaf pan with parchment paper.
- Then separate the egg whites and the yolks.
- Combine egg whites and cream of tartar in a large bowl. Then whip until stiff peaks form using a hand mixer.
- Beat yolks with melted butter, almond flour, baking powder, and salt in a separate large bowl using a hand mixer.
- Fold in ⅓ of the whipped egg whites until it is fully incorporated, then fold in the rest.
- Then pour batter into loaf pan and smooth top.
- Bake it for 30 minutes, or until top is slightly golden and toothpick inserted comes out clean.
- Let it cool 30 minutes before slicing.

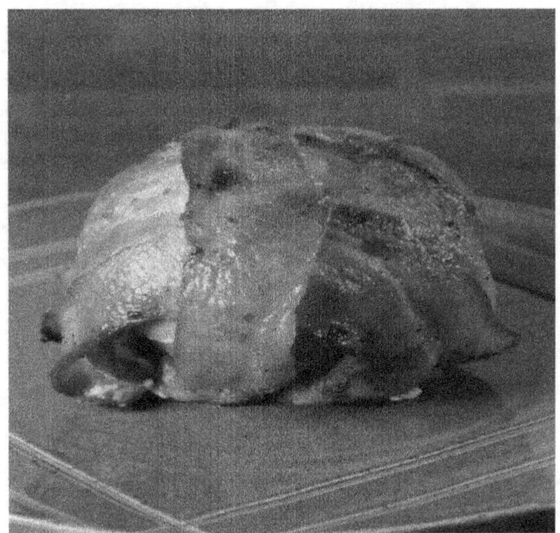
Bacon Avocado Bombs

INGREDIENTS

- 2 avocados
- ⅓ c. shredded Cheddar
- 8 slices bacon

PREPARATIONS

- First heat broiler and then line a small baking sheet with foil.
- Slice each of the avocado in half and remove the pits.
- Then peel the skin off of each avocado.
- Fill two of the halves with cheese, then replace with the other avocado halves.
- Wrap each of the avocado with 4 slices of bacon.
- Place bacon-wrapped avocados on the prepared baking sheet and broil until the bacon is crispy on top, about 5 minutes.
- Very carefully, flip the avocado using tongs and continue to cook until crispy all over, about 5 minutes per side.
- Cut into half crosswise and serve immediately.

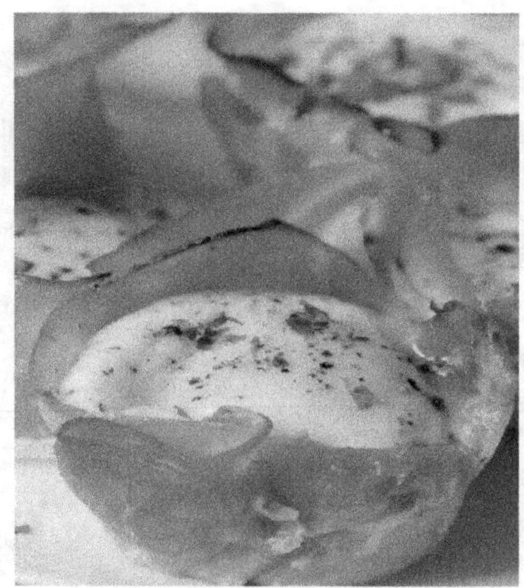

Ham & Cheese Egg Cups

INGREDIENTS

- Cooking spray, for pan
- 12 slices ham
- 1 c. shredded cheddar
- 12 large eggs
- kosher salt
- Freshly ground black pepper
- Chopped fresh parsley, for garnish

PREPARATIONS

- Preheat the oven to 400º and then grease a 12-cup muffin tin with cooking spray.
- After that, line each cup with a slice of ham and sprinkle with cheddar.
- Crack an egg into each ham cup and season with salt and pepper.
- Bake the eggs until they are cooked through, 12 to 15 minutes (depending on how runny you like your yolks).
- Garnish it with parsley and serve.

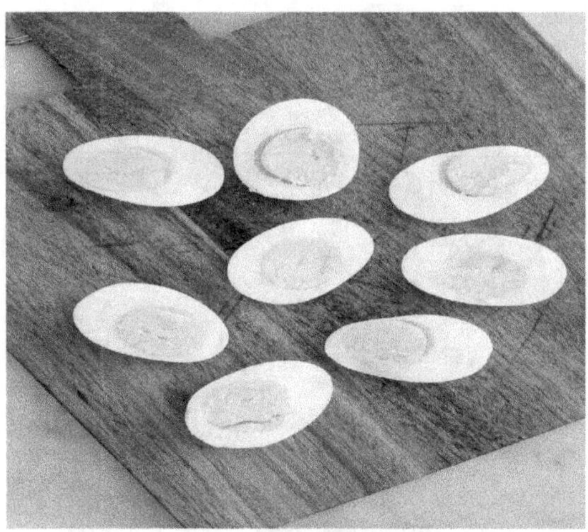

Hard Boil Eggs

INGREDIENTS

- 12 large eggs
- water

PREPARATIONS

- Place the eggs in a large pot and cover them with an inch of cold water.
- Then place the pot on the stove and bring to a boil.
- Instantly turn off heat and cover pot.
- Let sit for 11 minutes.
- Remove it from the pan and dunk it into ice water.
- Peel and serve.

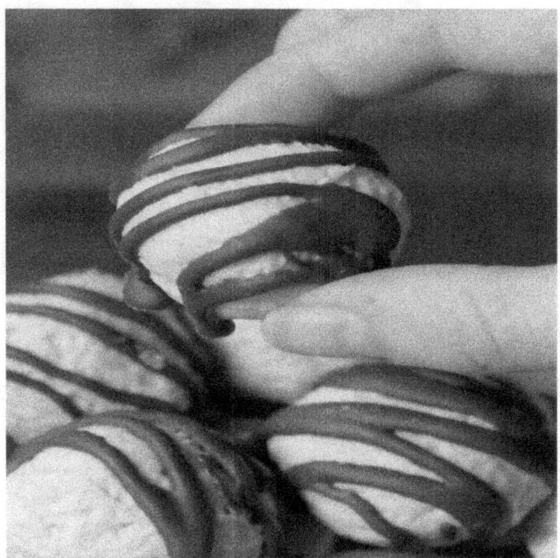

Keto Fat Bombs

INGREDIENTS

- 8 cream cheese, softened to room temperature
- ½ keto-friendly peanut butter
- ¼ coconut oil, plus 2 tbsp.
- ¼ tablespoon of kosher salt
- ½ keto-friendly dark chocolate chips

PREPARATIONS

- Firstly, line up a small baking sheet with parchment paper.
- In a medium bowl, combine cream cheese, peanut butter, ¼ cup coconut oil, and salt.
- Beat mixture until fully combined, about 2 minutes using a hand mixer.
- Place the bowl in the freezer to firm up slightly from 10 to 15 minutes.
- When the peanut butter mixture is hardened, use a small cookie scoop or spoon to create tablespoon-sized balls.
- Then place it in the refrigerator to harden, 5 minutes.

- Meanwhile, make chocolate drizzle: combine chocolate chips and remaining coconut oil in a microwave safe bowl and microwave in 30 second intervals until fully melted.
- Drizzle over peanut butter balls and place back in the refrigerator to harden, 5 minutes.
- To store, keep covered in the refrigerator.

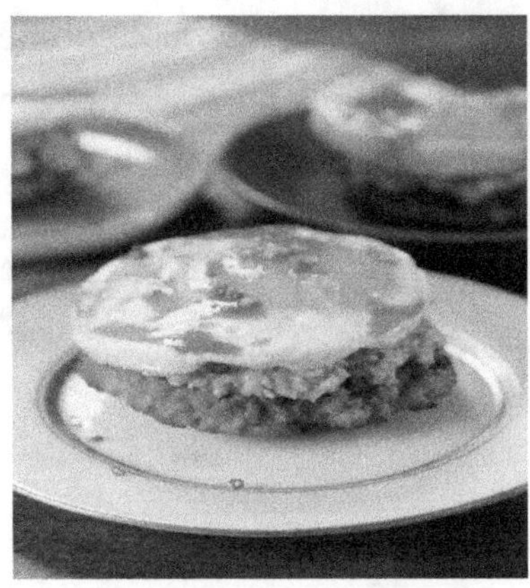

Paleo Breakfast Stacks

INGREDIENTS

- Three sausage patties (breakfast)
- One avocado mashed
- Kosher salt
- Freshly ground black pepper
- Three large eggs
- Chives, for garnish
- Hot sauce.

PREPARATIONS

- Heat the breakfast sausage according to the instructions on the box.
- Then mash the avocado into breakfast sausage and season it with salt and pepper.
- Then spray a medium skillet over medium heat with cooking spray
- Then spray the inside of the mason jar lid.
- Place mason jar lid in center of skillet and crack an egg inside.
- Season it with salt and pepper and let cook 3 minutes until whites are set, then remove the lid and continue cooking.
- Place egg on top of mashed avocado.
- Garnish with chives and drizzle with your favorite hot sauce.

The End

Thanks for taking the time to read my book. I hope it helped you out in some type of way. If you are not already please go now and follow me here on FB at

https://www.facebook.com/RichardRobertson40/ .

By following me you will receive updates on all of my upcoming books, giveaways, also you will be the first to get free copies of all of my books.

Never miss another update

You can also follow me here on my Author's Page on Amazon.

Just Because

Just because you took the time to read my book here are two of my Keto Diet Books **FREE**. Sign up and get your books.

<u>The guide to staying healthy after 40 for women...The Keto way</u>

<u>Staying fit after 40</u>